AIR FRYER

COOKBOOK FOR BEGINNERS

SNACK RECIPES

Quick, Easy and Tasty Recipes
for Smart People on a Budget

Nancy Johnson

Copyright © 2021 by Nancy Johnson

Legal Disclaimer

The information contained in this book and its contents is not designed to replace any form of medical or professional advice; and is not meant to replace the need for independent medical, financial, legal, or other professional advice or service that may require. The content and information in this book have been provided for educational and entertainment purposes only.

The content and information contained in this book have been compiled from sources deemed reliable, and they are accurate to the best of the Author's knowledge, information and belief.

However, the Author cannot guarantee its accuracy and validity and therefore cannot be held liable for any errors and/or omissions.

Further, changes are periodically made to this book as needed. Where appropriate and/or necessary, you must consult a professional (including but not limited to your doctor, attorney, financial advisor, or other such professional) before using any of the suggested remedies, techniques, and/or information in this book.

Upon using this book's contents and information, you agree to hold harmless the Author from any damaged, costs and expenses, including any legal fees potentially resulting from the application of any of the information in this book. This disclaimer applies to any loss, damages, or injury caused by the use and application of this book's content, whether directly and indirectly, whether for breach of contract, tort, negligence, personal injury, criminal intent, or under any other circumstances.

You agree to accept all risks of using the information presented in this book. You agree that by continuing to read this book, where appropriate and/or necessary, you shall consult a professional (including but not limited to your doctor, attorney, financial advisor, or other such professional) before remedies, techniques, and/or information in this book.

TABLE OF CONTENTS

AIR FRYER COOKBOOK: SNACK RECIPES

.

1. Tasty Baked Eggs

Prep Time20 mins | Serving 4 | Easy

INGREDIENTS:

- ➢ 4 eggs
- ➢ 1-pound of torn baby spinach
- ➢ 7 ounces of chopped ham
- ➢ 4 tablespoons of milk
- ➢ 1 tablespoon of olive oil
- ➢ Cooking spray
- ➢ Salt and black pepper to the taste

DIRECTIONS:

1. Prepare a pan of oil over medium pressure, add baby spinach, cook, and simmer for a few minutes.

2. Put cooking spray in 4 ramekins, add the baby spinach, ham, and break an egg in each of them.

3. Season with salt and pepper. Put bread in each ramekin. Put ramekins on preheated AirFryer at 350° F for twenty minutes.

Nutrition: Calories: 321, Fat: 6 g, Fiber: 8 g, Carbs: 15 g, Protein: 12 g.

2. Breakfast Egg Bowls

Prep Time20 mins | Serving 4 | Easy

INGREDIENTS:

➢ 4 dinner rolls, chopped the tops off, and scooped out the insides

➢ 4 tablespoons of heavy cream

➢ 4 eggs

➢ 4 teaspoons of chives mixed with parsley

➢ Salt and black pepper to taste

➢ 4 teaspoons of Parmesan

Instructions:

1. Arrange dinner rolls on a bakery tray and crack an egg in each.

2. Divide heavy cream, mixed herbs in each roll add salt and pepper to season.

3. Sprinkle your rolls with parmesan, put them in your air bowl and cook for 20 minutes at 350° F.

4. Divide between plates the bread bowls.

Enjoy!

Nutrition: Calories: 238, Fat: 4 g, Fiber: 7 g, Carbs: 14 g, Protein: 7 g.

3. Delicious Breakfast Soufflé

Prep Time16 mins | Serving 2 | Easy

INGREDIENTS:

➢ 4 eggs, whisked

➢ 4 tablespoons of heavy cream

➢ A pinch of red chili pepper, crushed

➢ 2 tablespoons of parsley, chopped

➢ 2 tablespoons of chives, chopped

➢ Salt and black pepper to the taste

DIRECTIONS:

1. Mix the eggs with salt, pepper, heavy cream, red chili pepper, parsley, chives in a pot, stir well, and split into 4 dishes of soufflé.

2. Arrange dishes in the AirFryer and cook the soufflés for 8 minutes at 350° F.

3. Serve them.

Enjoy!

Nutrition: Calories: 300, Fat: 7 g, Fiber: 9 g, Carbs: 15 g, Protein: 6 g.

4. Air Fried Sandwich

Prep Time16 mins | Serving 2 | Easy

INGREDIENTS:

➢ 2 English muffins halved

➢ 2 eggs

➢ 2 bacon strips

➢ Salt and black pepper to the taste

DIRECTIONS:

1. Crack eggs in your AirFryer, put bacon on top, cover, and cook at 392° F for 6 minutes.

2. Warm up the English muffin halves in the microwave for a few seconds, split eggs into two halves, place bacon on top, sprinkle salt and pepper, cover with the other two English muffins and serve for breakfast.

Enjoy!

Nutrition: Calories: 261, Fat: 5 g, Fiber: 8 g, Carbs: 12 g, Protein: 4 g.

5. Rustic Breakfast

Prep Time16 mins | Serving 2 | Easy

INGREDIENTS:

- 7 ounces baby spinach
- 8 chestnuts mushrooms, halved
- 8 tomatoes, halved
- 1 garlic clove, minced
- 4 chipolatas
- 4 bacon slices, chopped
- Salt and black pepper to the taste
- 4 eggs
- Cooking spray

DIRECTIONS:

1. Put the cooking spray over a frying pan and add onions, garlic, and mushrooms.

2. Add bacon and chipolatas, and finish with spinach and crack eggs.

3. Season with salt and pepper, bring the pan into the cooking basket of your AirFryer, and cook at 350° F for 13 minutes.

4. Serve for breakfast.**Nutrition:** Calories: 312, Fat: 6 g, Fiber:8 g, Carbs: 15 g, Protein: 5 g.

6. Egg Muffins

Prep Time25 mins | Serving 1 | Easy

INGREDIENTS:

- ➢ 1 egg
1. 2 tablespoons of olive oil
2. 3 tablespoons of milk
3. 3.5 ounces of white flour
4. 1 tablespoon of baking powder
5. 2 ounces of parmesan, grated
6. A splash of Worcestershire sauce
7. 1 tablespoon of starch
8. 2 tablespoon of butter

DIRECTIONS:

1. Mix the egg and starch, butter, baking powder, cheese, and parmesan in a pot, stir well, and split into 4 cups of silicon muffin.

2. Arrange cups in the cooking basket of your AirFryer, cover, and cook at 392° F for 15 minutes.

3. Serve warm.

Enjoy!

Nutrition: Calories: 251, Fat: 6g, Fiber: 8g, Carbs: 9g, Protein: 3g.

7. Polenta Bites

Prep Time30 mins | Serving 4 | Normal)

INGREDIENTS:

For the polenta:

- ➢ 1 tablespoon of butter
- ➢ 1 cup of cornmeal
- ➢ 3 cups of water
- ➢ Salt and black pepper to the taste

For the polenta bites:

- ➢ 2 tablespoons of powdered sugar
- ➢ Cooking spray

DIRECTIONS:

1. Mix water in a saucepan with cornmeal, sugar, salt, and pepper, stir, bring to a boil over medium heat, simmer for 10 minutes, take off heat, whisk again and hold in the refrigerator until it is cool.

2. Scoop 1 spoonful of polenta, shap

e a ball and place it on a working surface.

3. Repeat with the rest of the polenta, place all the balls in the cooking basket of your AirFryer, sprinkle them with cooking oil, cover, and steam for 8 minutes at 380° F.

4. Arrange bits of polenta on bowls, scatter sugar all over, and serve as toast.

Enjoy!

Nutrition: Calories: 231, Fat: 7g, Fiber: 8g, Carbs: 12g, Protein: 4g.

8 Delicious Breakfast Potatoes

Prep Time30 mins | Serving 4 | Normal)

INGREDIENTS:

- ➢ 2 tablespoons of olive oil
- ➢ 3 potatoes, cubed
- ➢ 1 yellow onion, chopped
- ➢ 1 red bell pepper, chopped
- ➢ Salt and black pepper to taste
- ➢ 1 teaspoon of garlic powder
- ➢ 1 teaspoon of sweet paprika
- ➢ 1 teaspoon of onion powder

DIRECTIONS:

1. Grease the basket of your AirFryer with olive oil, add the potatoes, mix with salt and pepper to season.

2. Combine onion, bell pepper, garlic powder, paprika, and onion powder, then mix properly, cover, and simmer for 30 minutes at 370° F.

3. Place potatoes on plates and serve as a snack.

Nutrition: Calories: 214, Fat: 6 g, Fiber: 8 g, Carbs: 15 g, Protein: 4 g.

9 Tasty Cinnamon Toast

(Preparation time: 10 min | Cooking time: 5 min | Servings: 6)

INGREDIENTS:

➢ 1 stick of butter, soft

➢ 12 bread slices

➢ ½ cup of sugar

➢ 1½ teaspoon of vanilla extract

➢ 1 ½ teaspoon of cinnamon powder

DIRECTIONS:

1. Mix the soft butter, the honey, and cinnamon in a cup and whisk well.

2. Spread this on the slices of bread, put them in your fryer, and cook at 400° F for 5 minutes.

3. Split between dishes and serve for breakfast.

Enjoy!

Nutrition: Calories: 221, Fat: 4 g, Fiber: 7 g, Carbs: 12 g, Protein: 8 g.

10. Delicious Potato Hash

Prep Time30 mins | Serving 4 | Normal)

INGREDIENTS:

- ➢ 1 ½ potatoes, cubed
- ➢ 1 yellow onion, chopped
- ➢ 2 teaspoons of olive oil
- ➢ 1 green bell pepper, chopped
- ➢ Salt and black pepper to the taste
- ➢ ½ teaspoon of dried thyme
- ➢ 2 eggs

DIRECTIONS:

1. Heat the AirFryer at 350° F, add oil, heat it, bell pepper, salt, and black pepper, stir and cook for 5 minutes.

2. Add the onions, thyme, and peas. Stir, cover, and simmer at 360° F for 20 minutes

3. Serve for breakfast.

Enjoy!

Nutrition: Calories: 241, Fat: 4 g, Fiber: 7 g, Carbs: 12 g, Protein: 7 g.

11. Sweet Breakfast Casserole

Prep Time40 mins | Serving 4 | Normal)

INGREDIENTS:

- ➢ 3 tablespoons of brown sugar
- ➢ 4 tablespoons of butter
- ➢ 2 tablespoons of white sugar
- ➢ ½ teaspoon cinnamon powder
- ➢ ½ cup flour
- ➢ For the casserole:
- ➢ 2 eggs
- ➢ 2 tablespoons of white sugar
- ➢ 2 ½ cups white flour
- ➢ 1 teaspoon of baking soda
- ➢ 1 teaspoon of baking powder
- ➢ 2 eggs
- ➢ ½ cup of milk
- ➢ 2 cups of buttermilk
- ➢ 4 tablespoons of butter
- ➢ Zest from 1 lemon, grated
- ➢ 1 2/3 cup blueberries

DIRECTIONS:

1. Mix the beans in a bowl of 2 tablespoons of white sugar, 2 and 1/2 cups of white flour, baking powder, baking soda, 2 potatoes, milk, buttermilk, 4 tablespoons of butter, lemon zest, and blueberries, stir and put into a saucepan that suits the fryer.

2. Mix 3 tablespoons of brown sugar with 2 tablespoons of white sugar, 4 tablespoons of butter, 1/2 cup of flour, and cinnamon in another dish, stir until a crumble is formed, and pour over the blueberries. Add ½ glass of milk.

3. Place in a preheated AirFryer and bake at 300° F for 30 minutes.

4. Serve for breakfast and split between dishes. Use olive oil for seasoning.

Enjoy!

Nutrition: Calories: 214, Fat: 5 g, Fiber: 8 g, Carbs: 12 g, Protein: 5 g.

12. Eggs Casserole

Prep Time30 mins | Serving 6 | Normal)

INGREDIENTS:

➢ 1-pound turkey, ground

➢ 1 tablespoon of olive oil

➢ ½ teaspoon of chili powder

➢ 12 eggs

➢ 1 sweet potato, cubed

➢ 1 cup of baby spinach

➢ Salt and black pepper to the taste

➢ 2 tomatoes, chopped for serving

DIRECTIONS:

1. Mix the eggs in a dish of salt, pepper, chili powder, spinach, sweet potato, and turkey, and whisk well.

2. At 350° F, heat your AirFryer, add oil, and heat it.

3. Attach a combination of eggs, scatter over your AirFryer, cover, and steam for 25 minutes.

4. Serve for breakfast and split between dishes.

Enjoy!

Nutrition: Calories: 300, Fat: 5 g, Fiber: 8 g, Carbs: 13 g, Protein: 6 g.

13. Sausage, Eggs, and Cheese Mix

Prep Time30 mins | Serving 4 | Normal)

INGREDIENTS:

➢ 10 ounces of sausages, cooked and crumbled

➢ 1 cup of cheddar cheese, shredded

➢ 1 cup of mozzarella cheese, shredded

➢ 8 eggs, whisked

➢ 1 cup of milk

➢ Salt and black pepper to the taste

➢ Cooking spray

DIRECTIONS:

1. Mix the sausages in a bowl with the cheese, mozzarella, eggs, milk, salt, and whisk well and add pepper.

2. Put cooking spray to the AirFryer and heat to 380° F, add the eggs, mix the bacon, and cook for about 20 minutes.

3. Divide into portions and serve.

Enjoy!

Nutrition: Calories: 320, Fat: 6 g, Fiber: 8 g, Carbs: 12 g, Protein: 5 g.

14. Cheese Air Fried Bake

Prep Time30 mins | Serving 4 | Normal)

INGREDIENTS:

➢ 4 bacon slices, cooked and crumbled

➢ 2 cups of milk

➢ 2 and ½ cups of cheddar cheese, shredded

➢ 1-pound breakfast sausage, casings removed and chopped

➢ 2 eggs

➢ ½ teaspoon of onion powder

➢ Salt and black pepper to the taste

➢ 3 tablespoons of parsley, chopped

➢ Cooking spray

DIRECTIONS:

1. Mix eggs in a bowl with milk, cheese, onion powder, salt, pepper, and parsley, then whisk well.

2. Grease your AirFryer with cooking spray, heat it to 320° F, and add bacon and sausage.

3. Attach mixture of the eggs, scatter and simmer for 20 minutes. Divide between plates.

Nutrition: Calories: 214, Fat: 5g, Fiber: 8g, Carbs: 12g, Protein: 12g.

15. Biscuits Casserole

Prep Time30 mins | Serving 8 | Normal)

INGREDIENTS:

- ➤ 12 ounces of biscuits, quartered
- ➤ 3 tablespoons of flour
- ➤ ½ pound of sausage, chopped
- ➤ A pinch of salt and black pepper
- ➤ 1 tablespoon of butter
- ➤ ½ cup rice
- ➤ 2 bacon strips
- ➤ 2 ½ cups of milk
- ➤ Cooking spray

DIRECTIONS:

1. Grease the AirFryer with cooking spray and pump it above 350° F.

2. At the edge, incorporate biscuits and blend with bacon.

3. Add the rice, butter, salt, and pepper, mix and cook for 15 minutes.

4. Serve for breakfast and split between dishes.

Enjoy!

Nutrition: Calories: 321, Fat: 4g, Fiber: 7g, Carbs: 12g, Protein: 5g.

16. Turkey Burrito

Prep Time20 mins | Serving 2 | Easy

INGREDIENTS:

- ➢ 4 slices of turkey breast already cooked
- ➢ ½ red bell pepper, sliced
- ➢ 2 eggs
- ➢ 1 small avocado, peeled, pitted, and sliced
- ➢ 2 tablespoons of parsley
- ➢ Salt and black pepper to the taste
- ➢ 1/8 cup mozzarella cheese, grated
- ➢ Tortillas for serving

DIRECTIONS:

1. Whisk eggs to taste in a bowl of salt and pepper, pour them into a saucepan, and put them in the AirFryer basket.

2. Cook at 400° F for 5 minutes, remove the saucepan from the fryer and switch eggs to a tray.

3. Arrange tortillas on a working board, spread eggs over them, spread turkey meat, bell pepper, cheese, salsa, and avocado as well.

4. Roll out your burritos and put them in your AirFryer after lining it with some tin foil.

5. Steam the burritos up at 300° F for 3 minutes, break them on plates and serve.

Enjoy!

Nutrition: Calories: 349, Fat: 23 g, Fiber: 11 g, Carbs: 20 g, Protein: 21 g.

17. Tofu Scramble

Prep Time30 mins | Serving 4 | Easy

INGREDIENTS:

- 2 tablespoons of soy sauce
- 1 tofu block, cubed
- 1 teaspoon of turmeric, ground
- 2 tablespoons of extra virgin olive oil
- 4 cups of broccoli florets
- ½ teaspoon of onion powder
- ½ teaspoon of garlic powder
- 2 and ½ cup of red potatoes, cubed
- ½ cup of yellow onion, chopped
- Salt and black pepper to the taste

DIRECTIONS:

1. In a cup, whisk and set aside to blend tofu with 1 tablespoon of butter, salt, pepper, soy sauce, garlic powder, onion powder, turmeric, and onion.

2. Combine potatoes with remaining oil in a separate dish, a sprinkle of salt and pepper, and mix to cover.

3. At 350° F, put the potatoes in your AirFryer and bake for 15 minutes, shaking once.

4. Attach marinade tofu to AirFryer and bake for about 15 minutes.

5. Attach broccoli to the fryer, and cook for another 5 minutes.

6. Serve forthwith.

Enjoy!

Nutrition: Calories: 140, Fat: 4 g, Fiber: 3 g, Carbs: 10 g, Protein: 14 g.

18. Oatmeal Casserole

Prep Time30 mins | Serving 8 | Easy

INGREDIENTS:

- 2 cups of rolled oats
- 1 teaspoon of baking powder
- 1/3 cup of brown sugar
- 1 teaspoon of cinnamon powder
- ½ cup of chocolate chips
- 2/3 cup of blueberries
- 1 banana, peeled and mashed
- 2 cups of milk
- 1 egg
- 2 tablespoons of butter
- 1 teaspoon of vanilla extract
- Cooking spray

DIRECTIONS:

1. Mix the sugar and baking powder, cinnamon, chocolate chips, blueberries, and banana in a bowl and stir.

2. Mix eggs with vanilla extract and butter in a separate cup, then whisk.

3. Heat up the AirFryer to 320° F, cook spray grease, and add oats to the rim.

4. Add the mixture of cinnamon and the eggs, toss, and cook for 20 minutes.

5. Stir once more, split into bowls, and serve breakfast.

Enjoy!

Nutrition: Calories: 300, Fat: 4 g, Fiber: 7 g, Carbs: 12 g, Protein: 10 g.

19. Ham Breakfast

Prep Time30 mins | Serving 6 | Easy

INGREDIENTS:

- ➢ 6 cups of French bread, cubed
- ➢ 4 ounces of green chilies, chopped
- ➢ 10 ounces of ham, cubed
- ➢ 4 ounces of cheddar cheese, shredded
- ➢ 2 cups of milk
- ➢ 5 eggs
- ➢ 1 tablespoon of mustard
- ➢ Salt and black pepper to the taste
- ➢ Cooking spray

DIRECTIONS:

1. Heat your AirFryer at 350° F and add cooking spray to grease it.

2. Mix the eggs in a bowl with the butter, cheese, mustard, salt, pepper, and whisk.

3. In your AirFryer, add the bread cubes and blend with the chilies and bacon.

4. Add the eggs, scatter over and simmer for 15 minutes.

5. Divide between plates.

Enjoy!

Nutrition: Calories: 200, Fat: 5g, Fiber: 6g, Carbs: 12g, Protein: 14g.

20. Tomato and Bacon Breakfast

Prep Time40 mins | Serving 6 | Normal)

INGREDIENTS:

- ➢ 1-pound of white bread, cubed
- ➢ 1-pound of smoked bacon, cooked and chopped
- ➢ ¼ cup of olive oil
- ➢ 1 yellow onion, chopped
- ➢ 28 ounces of canned tomatoes, chopped
- ➢ ½ teaspoon of red pepper, crushed
- ➢ ½ pound of cheddar, shredded
- ➢ 2 tablespoons of chives, chopped
- ➢ ½ pound of Monterey Jack, shredded
- ➢ 2 tablespoons of stock
- ➢ Salt and black pepper to the taste
- ➢ 8 eggs, whisked

DIRECTIONS:

1. Apply the oil to the AirFryer and heat at 350° F.

2. Add the bread, ham, cabbage, tomatoes, red pepper, and stir. Reserve.

3. Add bacon, cheddar, and Monterey jack and simmer for 20 minutes.

4. Divide between bowls, scatter with the chives and serve.

Enjoy!

Nutrition: Calories: 231, Fat: 5 g, Fiber: 7 g, Carbs: 12 g, Protein: 4 g.

21. Tasty Hash

Prep Time30 mins | Serving 6 | Easy

INGREDIENTS:

- ➢ 16 ounces of hash browns
- ➢ ¼ cup of olive oil
- ➢ ½ teaspoon of paprika
- ➢ ½ teaspoon of garlic powder
- ➢ Salt and black pepper to the taste
- ➢ 1 egg, whisked
- ➢ 2 tablespoon of chives, chopped
- ➢ 1 cup of cheddar, shredded

DIRECTIONS:

1. Apply the oil to the AirFryer, pump it up at 350° F, and apply brown hash.

2. Combine the paprika, garlic powder, salt, pepper, and egg, mix for 15 minutes, and fry.

3. Add the cheddar and chives, toss, break and serve between plates.

Enjoy!

Nutrition: Calories: 213, Fat: 7 g, Fiber: 8 g, Carbs: 12 g, Protein: 4 g.

22. Creamy Hash Browns

Prep Time30 mins | Serving 6 | Easy

INGREDIENTS:

- ➢ 2 pounds of browns hash
- ➢ 1 cup of whole milk
- ➢ 8 bacon slices, chopped
- ➢ 9 ounces of cream cheese
- ➢ 1 yellow onion, chopped
- ➢ 1 cup of cheddar cheese, shredded
- ➢ 6 green onions, chopped
- ➢ Salt and black pepper to the taste
- ➢ 6 eggs
- ➢ Cooking spray

DIRECTIONS:

1. Heat your AirFryer at 350° F and add cooking spray to grease it.

2. Combine eggs with butter, beans, cream cheese, cheddar cheese, bacon, onion, salt, pepper, and shake well into a dish.

3. Add hash browns to the AirFryer, start pouring the eggs over them and cook for 20 minutes.

4. Divide between plates and serve.

Enjoy!

Nutrition: Calories: 261, Fat: 6 g, Fiber: 9 g, Carbs: 8 g, Protein: 12 g.

23. Blackberry French Toast

Prep Time30 mins | Serving 4 | Easy

INGREDIENTS:

- 1 cup of blackberry jam, warm
- 12 ounces of bread loaf, cubed
- 8 ounces of cream cheese, cubed
- 4 eggs
- 1 teaspoon of cinnamon powder
- ½ cup of brown sugar
- 1 teaspoon of vanilla extract
- Cooking spray

DIRECTIONS:

1. Grease your AirFryer with cooking spray and heat it at 300° F.

2. Apply blueberry jam to the bottom, half the bread cubes on a plate, and apply cream cheese and finish with the rest of the crust.

3. Mix the eggs in a bowl of half and half, salt, sugar, and vanilla, stir well and pour the mixture to toast.

4. Cook for 20 minutes, divide between the dishes and serve for breakfast.

Enjoy!

Nutrition: Calories: 215, Fat: 6 g, Fiber: 9 g, Carbs: 16 g, Protein: 6 g.

24. Smoked Sausage Breakfast Mix

Prep Time40 mins | Serving 4 | Easy

INGREDIENTS:

- ➢ 1 and ½ pounds of smoked sausage, chopped and browned
- ➢ A pinch of salt and black pepper
- ➢ 1 and ½ cups of grits
- ➢ 4 and ½ cups of water
- ➢ 16 ounces of cheddar cheese, shredded
- ➢ 1 cup of milk
- ➢ ¼ teaspoon of garlic powder
- ➢ 1 and ½ teaspoons of thyme, chopped
- ➢ Cooking spray
- ➢ 4 eggs, whisked

DIRECTIONS:

1. Put the water in a kettle, over medium heat, bring to a boil, add grits, stir, cover, simmer for 5 minutes and take off the heat.

2. Stir the cheese, whisk until it melts, then blend well with the butter, thyme, salt, pepper, garlic powder, and eggs.

3. Heat the AirFryer at 300° F, grease with spray, and add pork sausage.

4. Stir in grits, scatter and simmer for 25 minutes.

5. Serve for breakfast and split between dishes.

Enjoy!

Nutrition: Calories: 321, Fat: 6 g, Fiber: 7 g, Carbs: 17 g, Protein: 4 g.

25. Delicious Potato Frittata

Prep Time30 mins | Serving 6 | Normal)

INGREDIENTS:

- ➢ 6 ounces of jarred roasted red bell peppers, chopped
- ➢ 12 eggs, whisked
- ➢ ½ cup of parmesan, grated
- ➢ 3 garlic cloves, minced
- ➢ 2 tablespoons of parsley, chopped
- ➢ Salt and black pepper to the taste
- ➢ 2 tablespoons of chives, chopped
- ➢ 16 potato wedges
- ➢ 6 tablespoons of ricotta cheese
- ➢ Cooking spray

DIRECTIONS:

1. Mix eggs in a bowl with red peppers, garlic, parsley, salt, pepper, and ricotta, then whisk well.

2. Heat the AirFryer at 300° F and apply cooking spray to oil it.

3. Add half of the potato wedges and sprinkle half of the parmesan over the bottom.

4. Add half the mixture of eggs, add the remaining potatoes, and the rest of the parmesan.

5. Remove the remaining blend of eggs, scatter the chives, and simmer for 20 minutes.

6. Serve for breakfast and split between dishes.

Enjoy!

Nutrition: Calories: 312, Fat: 6g, Fiber: 9g, Carbs: 16g, Protein: 5g.

26. Asparagus Frittata

Prep Time30 mins | Serving 2 | Easy

INGREDIENTS:

➤ 4 eggs, whisked

➤ 2 tablespoons of parmesan, grated

➤ 4 tablespoons of milk

➤ Salt and black pepper to the taste

➤ 10 asparagus tips, steamed

➤ Cooking spray

DIRECTIONS:

1. Mix the eggs with the parmesan, butter, salt, pepper, and whisk well in a pot.

2. Heat your AirFryer at 400° F and spray with grease.

3. Add asparagus, mix the eggs, toss a little, and cook for 5 minutes.

4. Split frittata into plates and serve for breakfast.

Enjoy!

Nutrition: Calories: 312, Fat: 5g, Fiber: 8g, Carbs: 14g, Protein: 2g.

27. Special Corn Flakes Breakfast Casserole

Prep Time18 mins | Serving 5 | Easy

INGREDIENTS:

- 1/3 cup of milk
- 3 teaspoons of sugar
- 2 eggs, whisked
- ¼ teaspoon of nutmeg, ground
- ¼ cup of blueberries
- 4 tablespoons of cream cheese, whipped
- 1 and ½ cups of corn flakes, crumbled
- 5 slices of bread

DIRECTIONS:

1. Mix the eggs and sugar, nutmeg, and milk in a bowl and whisk well.

2. Mix cream cheese with blueberries in another bowl and whisk well.

3. Place a single bowl of corn flakes.

4. Spread the blueberry mixture on each slice of bread, then mix in the eggs and dredge in the corn flakes at the end.

5. Place the bread in the basket of your AirFryer, set up at 400° F, and bake for 8 minutes.

6. Serve for breakfast and split between dishes.

Enjoy!

Nutrition: Calories: 300, Fat: 5g, Fiber: 7g, Carbs: 16g, Protein: 4g.

28. Ham Breakfast Pie

Prep Time35 mins | Serving 6 | Normal)

INGREDIENTS:

➢ 16 ounces of crescent rolls dough

➢ 2 eggs, whisked

➢ 2 cups of cheddar cheese, grated

➢ 1 tablespoon of parmesan, grated

➢ 2 cups of ham, cooked and chopped

➢ Salt and black pepper to the taste

➢ Cooking spray

DIRECTIONS:

1. Grease the pan of the AirFryer with a cooking spray and place half the dough on the bottom of the crescent rolls.

2. Mix eggs with cheddar cheese, parmesan, salt, and pepper in a bowl, whisk well, then add over dough.Place ham, spread the remaining crescent rolls in rows, place them over ham, and roast for 25 minutes at 300° F.

3. Pick pastry and serve for breakfast.

Nutrition: Calories: 400, Fat: 27 g, Fiber: 7 g, Carbs: 22 g, Protein: 16 g.

29. Breakfast Veggie Mix

Prep Time35 mins | Serving 6 | Normal)

INGREDIENTS:

- ➢ 1 yellow onion, sliced
- ➢ 1 red bell pepper, chopped
- ➢ 1 gold potato, chopped
- ➢ 2 tablespoons of olive oil
- ➢ 8 ounces of brie, trimmed and cubed
- ➢ 12 ounces of sourdough bread, cubed
- ➢ 4 ounces of parmesan, grated
- ➢ 8 eggs
- ➢ 2 tablespoons of mustard
- ➢ 3 cups of milk
- ➢ Salt and black pepper to the taste

DIRECTIONS:

1. At 350° F, heat up your AirFryer, add grease, onion, potato, and bell pepper and cook for 5 minutes.

2. Mix the eggs with sugar, salt, pepper, and mustard in a cup, then whisk well.

3. Add the bread and brie to the AirFryer, add half the mixture of the eggs, and add half the parmesan.

4. Add remaining bread and parmesan, toss just a bit and cook for 20 minutes.

5. Serve for breakfast and split between dishes.

Enjoy!

Nutrition: Calories: 231, Fat: 5 g, Fiber: 10 g, Carbs: 20 g, Protein: 12 g.

30. Scrambled Eggs

Prep Time20 mins | Serving 2 | Easy

INGREDIENTS:

- ➢ 2 eggs
- ➢ 2 tablespoons of butter
- ➢ Salt and black pepper to the taste
- ➢ 1 red bell pepper, chopped
- ➢ A pinch of sweet paprika

DIRECTIONS:

1. In a cup, mix salt, pepper, paprika, and red bell pepper with eggs, whisk well.

2. Heat the AirFryer at 140° F, and add melt butter.

3. Add the eggs, stir and simmer for 10 minutes.

4. Break scrambled eggs into plates, and it's done. Enjoy!

Nutrition: Calories: 200, Fat: 4 g, Fiber: 7 g, Carbs: 10 g, Protein: 3 g.

31. Fast Eggs and Tomatoes

Prep Time15 min | Servings 4 | Easy

INGREDIENTS:

➢ 4 eggs

➢ 2 ounces of milk

➢ 2 tablespoons of parmesan, grated

➢ Salt and black pepper to the taste

➢ 8 cherry tomatoes, halved

➢ Cooking spray

DIRECTIONS:

1. Grease the AirFryer with cooking spray and heat it at 200° F.

2. Mix the eggs in a cup with the cheese, butter, salt, pepper, and whisk.

3. Attach the mixture to the AirFryer and cook for 6 minutes.

4. Remove the tomatoes, cook the scrambled eggs for 3 minutes, split, and serve between plates.

Enjoy!

Nutrition: Calories: 200, Fat: 4 g, Fiber: 7 g, Carbs: 12 g, Protein: 3 g.

32. Air Fried Tomato Breakfast Quiche

Prep Time40 min | Servings 1 | Normal)

INGREDIENTS:

➢ 2 tablespoons of yellow onion, chopped

1. 2 eggs

2. ¼ cup of milk

3. ½ cup of gouda cheese, shredded

4. ¼ cup of tomatoes, chopped

5. Salt and black pepper to the taste

6. Cooking spray

DIRECTIONS:

1. Grease with cooking spray on a ramekin.

2. Crack eggs, stir and add cabbage, flour, sausages, milk, butter, cheese, tomatoes, salt, and pepper.

3. Put this in the pan of your AirFryer and cook for 30 minutes at 340° F.

4. Serve warm.

Enjoy!

Nutrition: Calories: 241, Fat: 6 g, Fiber: 8 g, Carbs: 14 g, Protein: 6 g.

33. Breakfast Mushroom Quiche

Prep Time20 min | Servings 4 | Normal)

INGREDIENTS:

- ➢ 1 tablespoon of flour
1. 1 tablespoon of butter, soft
2. 9-inch pie dough
3. 2 button of mushrooms, chopped
4. 2 tablespoons of ham, chopped
5. 3 eggs
6. A hand full of cabbage
7. ½ tablespoon butter
8. 1 small yellow onion, chopped
9. 1/3 cup of heavy cream
10. A pinch of nutmeg, ground
11. Salt and black pepper to the taste
12. ½ teaspoon of thyme, dried
13. ¼ cup of Swiss cheese, grated

DIRECTIONS:

1. Sift the flour on a working board, and roll the pastry dough.

2. Press your AirFryer on the bottom of the pie pan.

3. Mix butter and mushrooms, ham, cabbage, milk, heavy cream, cinnamon, pepper, thyme, nutmeg, and mix well in a pot.

4. Layer this over pie crust, scatter, spray all over Swiss cheese, and put pie pan in your AirFryer.

5. Cook the quiche for 10 minutes, at 400° F.

6. Slice to eat.

Enjoy!

Nutrition: Calories: 212, Fat: 4 g, Fiber: 6 g, Carbs: 7 g, Protein: 7 g.

34. Smoked Air Fried Tofu Breakfast

Prep Time22 min | Servings 2 | Normal)

INGREDIENTS:

➤ 1 tofu block, pressed and cubed

➤ Salt and black pepper to the taste

➤ 1 tablespoon of smoked paprika

➤ ¼ cup of cornstarch

➤ Cooking spray

DIRECTIONS:

1. Grease the basket from your AirFryer with cooking spray and heat the fryer to 370° F.

3. Mix tofu in a bowl with salt, pepper, smoked paprika, and cornstarch, then toss well.

3. Remove tofu to the AirFryer basket and cook every 4 minutes for 12 minutes, shaking the fryer.

4. Divide into plates.

Enjoy!

Nutrition: Calories: 172, Fat: 4 g, Fiber: 7 g, Carbs: 12 g, Protein: 4 g.

35. Delicious Tofu and Mushrooms

Prep Time20 min | Servings 2 | Easy

INGREDIENTS:

- ➤ 1 tofu block, pressed and cut into medium pieces
- ➤ 1 cup of panko bread crumbs
- ➤ Salt and black pepper to the taste
- ➤ ½ tablespoons of flour
- ➤ 1 egg
- ➤ 1 tablespoon of mushrooms, minced

DIRECTIONS:

1. Mix the egg with the mushrooms, flour, salt, and pepper in a bowl, then whisk well.

3. Dip the pieces of tofu in a mixture of eggs, then dredge them in crumbs of panko bread, put them in your AirFryer, and cook for 10 minutes at 350° F.

3. Serve them straight away for breakfast.

Enjoy!

Nutrition: Calories: 142, Fat: 4 g, Fiber: 6 g, Carbs: 8 g, Protein: 3 g.

36. Breakfast Broccoli Quiche

Prep Time30 min | Servings 2 | Normal)

INGREDIENTS:

- ➢ 1 broccoli head, florets separated, and steamed
- ➢ 1 tomato, chopped
- ➢ 3 carrots, chopped and steamed
- ➢ 2 ounces of cheddar cheese, grated
- ➢ 2 eggs
- ➢ 2 ounces of milk
- ➢ 1 teaspoon of parsley, chopped
- ➢ 1 teaspoon of thyme, chopped
- ➢ Salt and black pepper to the taste

DIRECTIONS:

1. Mix the eggs in a bowl with the milk, parsley, thyme, salt, pepper, and whisk well.

3. Place broccoli, tomato, and carrots in your AirFryer.

3. Add the eggs on top, spread the cheddar cheese, cover, and cook for 20 minutes at 350° F.

4. Serve for breakfast and split between dishes.

Enjoy!

Nutrition: Calories: 214, Fat: 4 g, Fiber: 7 g, Carbs: 12 g, Protein: 3 g.

37. Creamy Eggs

Prep Time22 min | Servings 4 | Easy

INGREDIENTS:

- ➢ 2 teaspoons of butter, soft
- ➢ 2 ham slices
- ➢ 4 eggs
- ➢ 2 tablespoons of heavy cream
- ➢ Salt and black pepper to the taste
- ➢ 3 tablespoons of parmesan, grated
- ➢ 2 teaspoons of chives, chopped
- ➢ A pinch of smoked paprika

DIRECTIONS:

1. Grease with butter the pan of your AirFryer, line it with the ham, and add it to the tray of your AirFryer.

3. Add 1 egg with heavy cream, salt, and pepper in a cup, then whisk well and pour over ham.

3. Crack the remaining eggs in the saucepan, sprinkle with parmesan, and cook your mix at 320° F for 12 minutes.Sprinkle all over the paprika and chives, and serve into plates.ù

Nutrition: Calories: 263, Fat: 5 g, Fiber: 8 g, Carbs: 12 g, Protein: 5 g.

38. Cheesy Breakfast Bread

Prep Time18 min | Servings 3 | Easy

INGREDIENTS:

➢ 6 bread slices

➢ 5 tablespoons of butter, melted

➢ 3 garlic cloves, minced

➢ 6 teaspoons of dried tomato pesto

➢ 1 cup of mozzarella cheese, grated

DIRECTIONS:

1. Arrange slices of bread on a working board.

2. Divide the tomato paste, garlic, and top with the grated cheese.

3. Attach slices of bread to your hot AirFryer, and cook for 8 minutes at 350° F.

4. Serve for breakfast and split between dishes.

Enjoy!

Nutrition: Calories: 187, Fat: 5 g, Fiber: 6 g, Carbs: 8 g, Protein: 3 g.

39. Breakfast Bread Pudding

Prep Time22 min | Servings 4 | Normal)

INGREDIENTS:

- ½ pound of white bread, cubed
- ¾ cup of milk
- ¾ cup of water
- 2 teaspoons of cornstarch
- ½ cup of apple, peeled, cored, and roughly chopped
- 5 tablespoons of honey
- 1 teaspoon of vanilla extract
- 2 teaspoons of cinnamon powder
- 1 and 1/3 cup of flour
- 3/5 cup of brown sugar
- 3 ounces of soft butter

DIRECTIONS:

1. Mix bread and apple in a cup, milk and sugar, butter, cinnamon, vanilla, and cornstarch, and whisk well.

3. Mix flour with sugar and butter in a separate bowl and stir until a crumbled mixture is obtained.

3. Place half the crumble mixes on the bottom of the AirFryer, add bread and apple mix, add the remainder of the crumble and cook for 22 minutes, all at 350° F.

4. Divide and serve the bread pudding in bowls.

Enjoy!

Nutrition: Calories: 261, Fat: 7 g, Fiber: 7 g, Carbs: 8 g, Protein: 5 g.

40. Buttermilk Breakfast Biscuits

Prep Time22 min | Servings 4 | Easy

INGREDIENTS:

➢ 1 ¼ cup of white flour

➢ ½ cup of self-rising flour

➢ ¼ teaspoon of baking soda

➢ ½ teaspoon of baking powder

➢ 1 teaspoon of sugar

➢ 4 tablespoons of butter, cold and cubed+ 1 tablespoon of melted butter

➢ ¾ cup of buttermilk

➢ Maple syrup for serving

DIRECTIONS:

1. Gather your INGREDIENTS: self-rising flour, baking soda, baking powder, unsalted butter and shortening, and buttermilk. Make sure everything is cold.

2. Add flour, butter, and shortening in a large bowl, and use a pastry cutter or your fingers to mix in butter and shortening.

3. Mix making a space in the middle of the bowl and pour in the buttermilk. Mix well.

4. Use a 2-inch biscuit cutter, flour it, and cut out biscuits. Place biscuits on AirFryer parchment sheet

liners (or a piece of parchment paper cut to fit your AirFryer) about 1 inch apart.

5. Air Fry on 400° Fahrenheit for 9 – 10 minutes and golden on top. Brush with melted butter and serve.

Enjoy!

Nutrition: Calories: 192, Fat: 6 g, Fiber: 9 g, Carbs: 12 g, Protein: 3 g.

41. Breakfast Bread Rolls

Prep Time22 min | Servings 4 | Easy

INGREDIENTS:

- ➤ 5 potatoes, boiled, peeled, and mashed
- ➤ 8 slices of bread, white parts only
- ➤ 1 coriander bunch, chopped
- ➤ 2 green chilies, chopped
- ➤ 2 small yellow onions, chopped
- ➤ ½ teaspoon of turmeric powder
- ➤ 2 curry leaf springs
- ➤ ½ teaspoon of mustard seeds
- ➤ 2 tablespoons of olive oil
- ➤ Salt and black pepper to the taste

DIRECTIONS:

1. Heat up a skillet with 1 tablespoon oil, add mustard seeds, onions, curry leaves, turmeric, stir a few seconds, and fry.

3. Add the mashed potatoes, salt, pepper, cilantro, and chilies, mix well, cook-off, and cool off.

3. Divide the potatoes into 8 pieces and use your wet hands to shape ovals.

4. Wet the slices of bread with water, click to remove excess water, and keep one slice in your hand.

5. Apply oval potato over a slice of bread and fold around it.

6. Continue for the remaining combination of potatoes and rolls.

7. Heat your AirFryer up at 400° F, add the remaining grease, add bread rolls and cook for 12 minutes.

8. Divide rolls of bread between plates and eat with tea for breakfast.

Enjoy!

Nutrition: Calories: 261, Fat: 6 g, Fiber: 9 g, Carbs: 12 g, Protein: 7 g.

42. Spanish Omelet

Prep Time20 min | Servings 4 | Normal)

INGREDIENTS:

➢ 3 eggs

- ½ chorizo, chopped

- 1 potato, peeled and cubed

- 1 medium head cabbage

- ½ cup milk

- 1 tablespoon cinnamon

- ½ cup of corn

- 1 tablespoon of olive oil

- 1 tablespoon of parsley, chopped

- 1 tablespoon of feta cheese, crumbled

- Salt and black pepper to the taste

DIRECTIONS:

1. Heat your AirFryer at 350° F, then add grease.

2. Stir in chorizo and onions, then brown for a few seconds.

3. Place the eggs in a dish with the corn, parsley, milk, salt, pepper, and whisk.

4. Pour over the chorizo and onions, scatter over them and cook for 5 minutes.

5. Cut omelet into plates and serve for breakfast.

Enjoy!

Nutrition: Calories: 300, Fat: 6 g, Fiber: 9 g, Carbs: 12 g, Protein: 6 g.

43. Egg White Omelet

Prep Time25 min | Servings 4 | Easy

INGREDIENTS:

- ➢ 1 cup of egg whites
- ➢ ¼ cup of tomato, chopped
- ➢ 2 tablespoons of skim milk
- ➢ ¼ cup of mushrooms, chopped
- ➢ 2 tablespoons of chives, chopped
- ➢ Salt and black pepper to the taste

DIRECTIONS:

1. Mix the egg whites with the tomato, milk, mushrooms, chives, salt, and pepper in a bowl, whisk well, and pour into the pan of your AirFryer.

2. Cook for 15 minutes at 320° F, cool down the omelet, break, split between the plates and eat.

Enjoy!

Nutrition: Calories: 100, Fat: 3 g, Fiber: 6 g, Carbs: 7 g, Carbs: 4 g.

44. Artichoke Frittata

Prep Time25 min | Servings 6 | Easy

INGREDIENTS:

➢ 3 canned artichokes hearts, drained and chopped

➢ 2 tablespoons of olive oil

➢ 1 chopped onion

➢ 1 cup milk

➢ ½ teaspoon of oregano, dried

➢ Salt and black pepper to the taste

➢ 6 eggs, whisked

DIRECTIONS:

1. Place the artichokes and the oregano, salt, pepper, feta cheese, and eggs in a bowl and whisk well.

3. Apply the oil to the pan of your AirFryer, blend with the eggs, and cook for 15 minutes at 320° F.

3. Cut frittata into plates and eat.

Enjoy!

Nutrition: Calories: 136, Fat: 6 g, Fiber: 6 g, Carbs: 9 g, Protein: 4 g.

45. Amazing Breakfast Burger

Prep Time55 min | Servings 4 | Normal)

INGREDIENTS:

- ➢ 1-pound beef, ground
- ➢ 1 yellow onion, chopped
- ➢ 1 teaspoon of tomato puree
- ➢ 1 teaspoon of garlic, minced
- ➢ 1 teaspoon of mustard
- ➢ 1 tablespoon ketchup
- ➢ 1 table spoon of mayonnaise
- ➢ 1 teaspoon of basil, dried
- ➢ 1 teaspoon of parsley, chopped
- ➢ 1 tablespoon of cheddar cheese, grated
- ➢ Salt and black pepper to the taste
- ➢ 4 bread buns, for serving

DIRECTIONS:

Make the sauce: In a small bowl, whisk together mayonnaise, ketchup, mustard, salt and pepper. Refrigerate until you're ready to assemble the burgers.

Make the burgers: Line a rimmed baking sheet with parchment paper and set aside. In a medium bowl, combine beef, sausage, Worcestershire sauce and garlic powder and season with salt and pepper. Using your hands, mix well. Shape into six 4-oz. patties that are about 4 inches in diameter and place them on the prepared baking sheet. Cover and refrigerate at least 30 minutes.

In a large cast-iron skillet or stovetop griddle over medium-high heat, heat 1 tablespoon oil. Remove burgers from the oven and cook three at a time, pressing with the back of a spatula, to your desired doneness—about 4 minutes per side for medium. In the last minute of cooking, top each patty with a slice of cheese. Transfer the burgers to a plate. Add remaining tablespoon oil to the pan and repeat with remaining patties.

Split the buns and spread both sides with sauce. Put cheeseburgers on the bottom halves of the buns, then top each with a fried egg, 2 bacon pieces, a slice of tomato, lettuce, and the top of the bun.

Nutrition: Calories: 234, Fat: 5 g, Fiber: 8 g, Carbs: 12 g, Protein: 4 g.

46. Onion Frittata

Prep Time30 min | Servings 6 | Easy

INGREDIENTS:

- ➢ 10 eggs, whisked
- ➢ 1 tablespoon of olive oil
- ➢ 1 tomato
- ➢ 2 carrots chopped
- ➢ 1-pound of small potatoes, chopped
- ➢ 2 yellow onions, chopped
- ➢ Salt and black pepper to the taste
- ➢ 1-ounce of cheddar cheese, grated
- ➢ ½ cup sour cream

DIRECTIONS:

1. Layer eggs with tomatoes, carrots, salt, pepper, potatoes, cheese, and saucepan in a wide bowl and whisk well.

2. Grease with oil the saucepan of your AirFryer, add the eggs, put in the AirFryer

And cook to 320° F for 20 minutes.

3. Slice the frittata, divide between the plates and serve as breakfast.

Enjoy!

Nutrition: Calories: 231, Fat: 5 g, Fiber: 7 g, Carbs: 8 g, Protein: 4 g.

47. Bell Peppers Frittata

Prep Time30 min | Servings 4 | Easy

INGREDIENTS:

➢ 2 tablespoons of olive oil

➢ ½ pounds of chicken sausage, casings removed and chopped

➢ 1 sweet onion, chopped

➢ 1 red bell pepper, chopped

➢ 1 orange bell pepper, chopped

➢ 1 green bell pepper, chopped

➢ Salt and black pepper to the taste

➢ 8 eggs, whisked

➢ ½ cup of mozzarella cheese, shredded

➢ 2 teaspoons of oregano, chopped

DIRECTIONS:

1. Add 1 spoonful of oil to the AirFryer, add bacon, heat to 320° F, and brown for 1 minute.

2. Mix the remaining, onion, red, orange and green bell pepper, and simmer for another 2 minutes.

3. Add oregano, salt, pepper, and eggs. Stir and cook for 15 minutes.

4. Add mozzarella, leave frittata aside for a couple of minutes, divide and serve between plates.

Enjoy!

Nutrition: Calories: 212, Fat: 4 g, Fiber: 6 g, Carbs: 8 g, Protein: 12 g.

48. Cheese Sandwich

Prep Time18 min | Servings 1 | Easy

INGREDIENTS:

➢ 2 bread slices

➢ 2 teaspoons of butter

➢ 2 pieces of cheddar cheese

➢ A pinch of sweet paprika

DIRECTIONS:

1. Place the butter on slices of bread, add the cheddar cheese on one, sprinkle the paprika, cover with the other slices of bread, break into 2 halves, put them in the AirFryer, and cook for 8 minutes at 370° F, turn them once, put them on a plate and serve.

Enjoy!

Nutrition: Calories: 130, Fat: 3 g, Fiber: 5 g, Carbs: 9 g, Protein: 3 g.

49. Long Beans Omelet

Prep Time20 min | Servings 3 | Easy

INGREDIENTS:

➢ ½ teaspoon of soy sauce

➢ 1 tablespoon of olive oil

➢ 3 eggs, whisked

➢ A pinch of salt and black pepper

➢ 4 garlic cloves, minced

➢ 4 long beans, trimmed and sliced

DIRECTIONS:

1. Mix the eggs in a bowl with a touch of salt, black pepper, and soy sauce, then whisk well.

4. At 320° F, heat up your AirFryer, add oil and garlic, stir, and brown for 1 minute.

3. Combine long beans and eggs, sprinkle and simmer for 10 minutes.

4. Break omelet into plates and serve for breakfast.

Enjoy!

Nutrition: Calories: 200, Fat: 3 g, Fiber: 7 g, Carbs: 9 g, Protein: 3 g.

50. French Beans and Egg Breakfast Mix

Prep Time20 min | Servings 3 | Easy

INGREDIENTS:

➢ 2 eggs, whisked

➢ ½ teaspoon of soy sauce

➢ 1 tablespoon of olive oil

➢ 4 garlic cloves, minced

➢ 3 ounces of French beans, trimmed and sliced diagonally

➢ Salt and white pepper to the taste

DIRECTIONS:

1. Mix the eggs with soy sauce, salt, and pepper in a bowl, then whisk properly.

2. Power the AirFryer up to 320° F, add oil, and fire it up too.

3. Add garlic and brown for 1 minute.

4. Stir French beans and egg mixture, toss for 10 minutes, then fry.

5. Serve for breakfast and split between dishes.

Enjoy!

Nutrition: Calories: 182, Fat: 3 g, Fiber: 6 g, Carbs: 8 g, Protein: 3 g.

51. Breakfast Doughnuts

Prep Time28 min | Servings 6 | Easy

INGREDIENTS:

➤ 4 tablespoons of butter, soft

➤ 1 and ½ teaspoon of baking powder

➤ 2 and ¼ cups of white flour

➤ ½ cup of sugar

➤ 1/3 cup of caster sugar

➤ 1 teaspoon of cinnamon powder

➤ 2 egg yolks

➤ ½ cup of sour cream

DIRECTIONS:

1. In a bowl, mix butter with simple sugar and egg yolks and well for 2 tablespoons.

4. Then add half the sour cream and stir.

3. Mix flour and baking powder in another bowl, stir and add to the mixture of eggs as well.

4. Stir well until a dough is obtained, transfer it onto a floured working surface, roll it out and cut large circles in the middle with smaller ones.

5. Brush the doughnuts with the remaining butter, heat your AirFryer at 360° F, place the doughnuts inside and cook for 8 minutes.

6. Mix the cinnamon and caster sugar in a bowl, and stir.

7. Arrange the doughnuts on plates, and before serving, dip them in cinnamon and sugar.

Enjoy!

Nutrition: Calories: 182, Fat: 3g, Fiber: 7g, Carbs: 8g, Protein: 3g.

52. Creamy Breakfast Tofu

Prep Time35 min | Servings 4 | Normal)

INGREDIENTS:

➢ 1 block of firm tofu, pressed and cubed

➢ 1 teaspoon of rice vinegar

➢ 2 tablespoons of soy sauce

➢ 2 teaspoons of sesame oil

➢ 1 tablespoon of potato starch

➢ 1 cup of Greek yogurt

DIRECTIONS:

1. Mix tofu cubes with vinegar, soy sauce, and oil in a bowl, toss and leave on for 15 minutes.

2. Dip tofu cubes into potato starch, toss, transfer to your AirFryer, heat up at 370° F, and cook halfway for 20 minutes.

3. Divide into bowls and serve with some Greek yogurt on the side for breakfast.

Enjoy!

Nutrition: Calories: 110, Fat: 4g, Fiber: 5g, Carbs: 8g, Protein: 4g.

53. Veggie Burritos

Prep Time20 min | Servings 4 | Easy

INGREDIENTS:

- ➢ 2 tablespoons of cashew butter
- ➢ 2 tablespoons of tamari
- ➢ 2 tablespoons of water
- ➢ 2 tablespoons of liquid smoke
- ➢ 4 rice papers
- ➢ ½ cup of sweet potatoes, steamed and cubed
- ➢ ½ small broccoli head, florets separated and steamed
- ➢ 7 asparagus stalks
- ➢ 8 roasted red peppers, chopped
- ➢ 1 kale, chopped

DIRECTIONS:

1. Mix cashew butter and water, tamari, and liquid smoke in a bowl, then whisk well.

4. Wet rice papers on a working surface and arrange them on.

3. Divide sweet potatoes, broccoli, asparagus, red peppers, kale, wrap burritos, and dip each into a mixture of cashews.

4. Arrange the burritos in the AirFryer and cook for 10 minutes at 350° F.

5. Divide veggie burritos on serving and serve for breakfast.

Enjoy!

Nutrition: Calories: 172, Fat: 4g, Fiber: 7g, Carbs: 8g, Protein: 3g.

54. Breakfast Fish Tacos

Prep Time23 min | Servings 4 | Normal)

INGREDIENTS:

➢ 4 big tortillas

1. 1 red bell pepper, chopped

2. 1 yellow onion, chopped

3. 1 cup of corn

4. 4 white fish fillets, skinless and boneless

5. ½ cup of salsa

6. A handful of mixed romaine lettuce, spinach, and radicchio

7. 4 tablespoon of parmesan, grated

DIRECTIONS:

1. Place the fish fillets in the AirFryer and cook for 6 minutes at 350° F.

2. In the meantime, prepare a casserole over medium heat, add bell pepper, onion, and corn, mix and simmer for 1-2 minutes.

3. Place tortillas on a working board, cut fish fillets, and scatter salsa. Divide mixed vegetables and mixed greens over them, then add parmesan at the end of each.

4. Roll your tacos, put them in the preheated AirFryer, and cook for another 6 minutes at 350° F.

5. Slice fish tacos into plates and eat for breakfast. Enjoy!

Nutrition: Calories: 200, Fat: 3g, Fiber: 7g, Carbs: 9g, Protein: 5g.

55. Garlic Potatoes with Bacon

Prep Time30 min | Servings 4 | Easy

INGREDIENTS:

➢ 4 potatoes, peeled and cut into medium cubes

1. 6 garlic cloves, minced

2. 4 bacon slices, chopped

3. 2 rosemary springs, chopped

4. 1 tablespoon of olive oil

5. Salt and black pepper to the taste

6. 2 eggs, whisked

DIRECTIONS:

1. Mix oil and onions, ginger, bacon, rosemary, cinnamon, pepper, and eggs and whisk in your AirFryer pan.

. Cook potatoes for 20 minutes at 400° F, put everything on plates, and serve as breakfasts.

Enjoy!

Nutrition: Calories: 211, Fat: 3g, Fiber: 5g, Carbs: 8g, Protein: 5g.

56. Spinach Breakfast Parcels

Prep Time14 min | Servings 2 | Normal)

INGREDIENTS:

- ➤ 4 sheets of filo pastry
- ➤ 1-pound of baby spinach leaves, roughly chopped
- ➤ ½ pound of ricotta cheese
- ➤ 2 tablespoons of pine nuts
- ➤ 1 egg, whisked
- ➤ Zest from 1 lemon, grated
- ➤ Greek yogurt for serving
- ➤ Salt and black pepper to the taste

DIRECTIONS:

1. Mix the spinach and cheese, egg, lemon zest, salt, pepper, and pine nuts in a bowl and stir.

2. Arrange filo sheets on a working board, split the spinach mixture, fold diagonally to form the parcels, and position them at 400° F in your preheated AirFryer.

3.Bake the packages for 4 minutes, split them into plates, and eat them sideways with Greek yogurt.

Enjoy!

Nutrition: Calories: 182, Fat: 4g, Fiber: 8g, Carbs: 9g, Protein: 5g.

57. Ham Rolls

Prep Time20 min | Servings 4 | Normal)

INGREDIENTS:

- ➢ 1 sheet of puff pastry
- ✓ 4 handful gruyere of cheese, grated
- ✓ 4 teaspoons of mustard
- ✓ 8 ham slices, chopped

DIRECTIONS:

1. On a flat surface, lay out the puff pastry, split the cheese, the ham, and mustard, close slice, and medium round break.

2. Put all rolls in AirFryer and cook at 370° F for 10 minutes.

3. Slice rolls on plates and serve.

Enjoy!

Nutrition: Calories: 182, Fat: 4g, Fiber: 7g, Carbs: 9g, Protein: 8g.

58. Shrimp Frittata

Prep time 25 min | Servings 4 | Normal

INGREDIENTS:

- 4 eggs
- ½ teaspoon of basil, dried
- Cooking spray
- Salt and black pepper to the taste
- ½ cup of rice, cooked
- ½ cup shrimp, cooked, peeled, deveined, and chopped
- ½ cup baby spinach, chopped
- ½ cup Monterey jack cheese, grated

DIRECTIONS:

1. In a bowl, mix eggs with salt, pepper, and basil and whisk.

2. Grease the pan of your AirFryer with cooking spray and add rice, shrimp, and spinach.

3. Add egg mix, sprinkle cheese all over, and cook in your AirFryer at 350° F for 10 minutes.

4. Divide among plates and serve for breakfast.

Enjoy!

Nutrition: Calories: 162, Fat: 6g, Fiber: 5g, Carbs: 8g, Protein: 4g.

59. Tuna Sandwiches

Prep time 15 min | Servings 4 | Easy

INGREDIENTS:

- 16 ounces of canned tuna, drained
- ¼ cup of mayonnaise
- 2 tablespoons of mustard
- 1 tablespoon of lemon juice
- 2 green onions, chopped
- 3 English muffins, halved
- 3 tablespoons of butter
- 6 provolone of cheese

DIRECTIONS:

1. In a bowl, mix tuna with mayo, lemon juice, mustard, and green onions and stir.

2. Grease muffin halves with the butter, place them in preheated AirFryer and bake them at 350° F for 4 minutes.

3. Spread tuna mix on muffin halves, top each with provolone cheese, return sandwiches to AirFryer and cook them for 4 minutes, divide among plates and serve for breakfast right away.

Enjoy!

Nutrition: Calories: 182, Fat: 4g, Fiber: 7g, Carbs: 8g, Protein: 6g.

60. Shrimp Sandwiches

Prep time 15 min | Servings 4 | Easy

INGREDIENTS:

➢ 1 and ¼ cups of cheddar, shredded

➢ 6 ounces of canned tiny shrimp, drained

➢ 3 tablespoons of mayonnaise

➢ 2 tablespoons of green onions, chopped

➢ 4 whole-wheat bread slices

➢ 2 tablespoons of butter, soft

DIRECTIONS:

1. Mix shrimp and cheese, green onion, and mayo in a cup, then mix well.

2. Place this over half of the slices of bread, cover with the other slices of bread, diagonally split into halves, and sprinkle butter over them.

3. Place the sandwiches in the AirFryer and cook for 5 minutes at 350° F.

4. Split shrimp on sandwiches and serve for breakfast.

Enjoy!

Nutrition: Calories: 162, Fat: 3g, Fiber: 7g, Carbs: 12g, Protein: 4g.

61. Breakfast Pea Tortilla

Prep Time 17 min | Servings 8 | Easy

INGREDIENTS:

- ½ pound of baby peas
- 4 tablespoons of butter
- 1 and ½ cup of yogurt
- 8 eggs
- ½ cup of mint, chopped
- Salt and black pepper to the taste

DIRECTIONS:

1. Heat a saucepan over medium heat that matches your AirFryer with the oil, add peas, stir and cook for a few minutes.

2. Meanwhile, mix half the yogurt with salt, pepper, eggs, and mint in a cup, then whisk well.

3. Pour over the peas, toss, stir in the AirFryer and cook for 7 minutes at 350° F.

4. Pour the remaining yogurt over the tortilla, peel, and serve.

Enjoy!

Nutrition: Calories: 192g, Fat: 5g, Fiber: 4g, Carbs: 8g, Protein: 7g.

62. Raspberry Rolls

Prep time 50 min | Servings 6 | Normal

INGREDIENTS:

- 1 cup of milk
- 4 tablespoons of butter
- 3 and ¼ cups of flour
- 2 teaspoons of yeast
- ¼ cup of sugar
- 1 egg

For the filling:

- 8 ounces of cream cheese, soft
- 12 ounces of raspberries
- 1 teaspoon of vanilla extract
- 5 tablespoons of sugar
- 1 tablespoon of cornstarch
- Zest from 1 lemon, grated

DIRECTIONS:

1. Mix the flour with the sugar and leaven in a bowl and whisk.

2. Attach milk and egg, stir until a dough is formed, set it aside for 30 minutes to rise, move the dough to a working surface, and roll well.

3. Mix cream cheese with butter, vanilla, and lemon zest in a cup, then stir well and scatter over bread.

4. Mix raspberries and cornstarch in another dish, stir and scatter over it. Combine cream cheese.

5. Shape your bread, break it into small parts, put it in your AirFryer, spray it with a cooking spray, and cook it for 30 minutes at 350° F.

6. Serve for breakfast.

Enjoy!

Nutrition: Calories: 261, Fat: 5g, Fiber: 8g, Carbs: 9g, Protein: 6g.

Potato and Leek Frittata

Prep time in about 28 min | Servings 4 | Normal

INGREDIENTS:

- ➢ 2 gold potatoes, boiled, peeled, and chopped
- ➢ 2 tablespoons of butter
- ➢ 2 leeks, sliced
- ➢ Salt and black pepper to the taste
- ➢ ¼ cup of whole milk
- ➢ 10 eggs, whisked
- ➢ 5 ounces of white cheese, crumbled

DIRECTIONS:

1. Heat a pan over medium heat that suits your AirFryer with the oil, add leeks, stir and cook for 4 minutes.

2. Attach the onions, salt, pepper, bacon, cheese, and butter, whisk well, cook for another 1 minute, put in AirFryer, and cook at 350° F for 13 minutes.

3. Break the frittata into cups, slice, and serve.

Enjoy!

Nutrition: Calories: 271, Fat: 6g, Fiber: 8g, Carbs: 12g, Protein: 6g.

64. Espresso Oatmeal

Prep time 27 min | Servings 4 | Normal

INGREDIENTS:

- ➢ 1 cup of milk
- ➢ 1 cup of steel-cut oats
- ➢ 2 and ½ cups of water
- ➢ 2 tablespoons of sugar
- ➢ 1 teaspoon of espresso powder
- ➢ 2 teaspoons of vanilla extract

DIRECTIONS:

1. Mix oats with tea, sugar, milk, and espresso powder in a saucepan that suits your AirFryer, stir, place in your AirFryer and cook for 17 minutes at 360° F.

2. Attach the vanilla extract, whisk, set all 5 minutes off, split into bowls and serve.

Enjoy!

Nutrition: Calories: 261, Fat: 7g, Fiber: 6g, Carbs: 39g, Protein: 6g.

65. Mushroom Oatmeal

Prep time 30 min | Servings 4 | Normal

INGREDIENTS:

- ➤ 1 small yellow onion, chopped
- ➤ 1 cup of steel-cut oats
- ➤ 2 garlic cloves, minced
- ➤ 2 tablespoons of butter
- ➤ ½ cup of water
- ➤ 14 ounces of canned chicken stock
- ➤ 3 thyme springs, chopped
- ➤ 2 tablespoons of extra virgin olive oil
- ➤ ½ cup of gouda cheese, grated
- ➤ 8 ounces of mushroom, sliced
- ➤ Salt and black pepper to the taste

DIRECTIONS

1. Heat a pan over medium heat that suits your AirFryer with the butter, add onions and garlic, stir and cook for 4 minutes.

2. Attach oats, sugar, salt, pepper, stock, and thyme, stir, place in the AirFryer and cook for 16 minutes at 360° F.

3. In the meantime, prepare a skillet over medium heat with the olive oil, add mushrooms, cook them

for 3 minutes, add oatmeal and cheese, whisk, divide into bowls and serve for breakfast.

Enjoy!

Nutrition: Calories: 284, Fat: 8g, Fiber: 8g, Carbs: 20g, Protein: 17g.

66. Walnuts and Pear Oatmeal

Prep time 17 min | Servings 4 | Normal

INGREDIENTS:

- ➤ 1 cup of water
- ➤ 1 tablespoon of butter, soft
- ➤ ¼ cups of brown sugar
- ➤ ½ teaspoon of cinnamon powder
- ➤ 1 cup of rolled oats
- ➤ ½ cup of walnuts, chopped
- ➤ 2 cups of pear, peeled and chopped
- ➤ ½ cup of raisins

DIRECTIONS:

1. Mix milk with honey, butter, oats, cinnamon, raisins, pears, and walnuts in a heat-proof dish that suits your AirFryer, stir, add into your fryer and cook for 12 minutes at 360° F.

2. Divide in and serve in pots.

Enjoy!

Nutrition: Calories: 230, Fat: 6g, Fiber: 11g, Carbs: 20g, Protein: 5g.

67. Cinnamon and Cream Cheese Oats

Prep time 35 min | Servings 4 | Normal

INGREDIENTS:

- ➢ 1 cup of steel oats
- ➢ 3 cups of milk
- ➢ 1 tablespoon of butter
- ➢ ¾ cup of raisins
- ➢ 1 teaspoon of cinnamon powder
- ➢ ¼ cup of brown sugar
- ➢ 2 tablespoons of white sugar
- ➢ 2 ounces of cream cheese, soft

Directions:

1. Heat a saucepan over medium heat that fits your AirFryer with the butter, add oats, stir and toast for 3 minutes.

2. Attach the milk and raisins, stir, place in the AirFryer and cook for 20 minutes at 350° F.

3. Meanwhile, mix cinnamon and brown sugar in a bowl, and stir.

4. Mix white sugar and cream cheese in a second bowl, then whisk.

5. Divide oats into bowls and top each with the cream cheese and cinnamon.

Enjoy!

Nutrition: Calories: 152, Fat: 6g, Fiber: 6g, Carbs: 25g, Protein: 7g.

CPSIA information can be obtained
at www.ICGtesting.com
Printed in the USA
BVHW090225060621
608544BV00015B/1531

9 781802 857399